T0254410

Cambridge Elements ≡

Elements of Improving Quality and Safety in Healthcare
edited by
Mary Dixon-Woods,[*] Katrina Brown,[*] Sonja Marjanovic,[†]
Tom Ling,[†] Ellen Perry,[*] and Graham Martin[*]
*THIS Institute (The Healthcare Improvement Studies Institute)
†RAND Europe

THE POSITIVE DEVIANCE APPROACH

Ruth Baxter[1] and Rebecca Lawton[1,2]

[1] Yorkshire Quality and Safety Research Group,
Bradford Institute for Health Research
[2] School of Psychology, University of Leeds

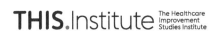
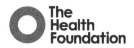

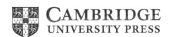

CAMBRIDGE
UNIVERSITY PRESS

CAMBRIDGE
UNIVERSITY PRESS

University Printing House, Cambridge CB2 8BS, United Kingdom

One Liberty Plaza, 20th Floor, New York, NY 10006, USA

477 Williamstown Road, Port Melbourne, VIC 3207, Australia

314–321, 3rd Floor, Plot 3, Splendor Forum, Jasola District Centre,
New Delhi – 110025, India

103 Penang Road, #05–06/07, Visioncrest Commercial, Singapore 238467

Cambridge University Press is part of the University of Cambridge.

It furthers the University's mission by disseminating knowledge in the pursuit of
education, learning, and research at the highest international levels of excellence.

www.cambridge.org
Information on this title: www.cambridge.org/9781009237116
DOI: 10.1017/9781009237130

© THIS Institute 2022

First published 2022

A catalogue record for this publication is available from the British Library.

ISBN 978-1-009-23711-6 Paperback
ISSN 2754-2912 (online)
ISSN 2754-2904 (print)

Cambridge University Press has no responsibility for the persistence or accuracy of
URLs for external or third-party internet websites referred to in this publication
and does not guarantee that any content on such websites is, or will remain,
accurate or appropriate.

Every effort has been made in preparing this Element to provide accurate and up-to-
date information that is in accord with accepted standards and practice at the time of
publication. Although case histories are drawn from actual cases, every effort has been
made to disguise the identities of the individuals involved. Nevertheless, the authors,
editors, and publishers can make no warranties that the information contained herein
is totally free from error, not least because clinical standards are constantly changing
through research and regulation. The authors, editors, and publishers therefore dis-
claim all liability for direct or consequential damages resulting from the use of material
contained in this Element. Readers are strongly advised to pay careful attention to
information provided by the manufacturer of any drugs or equipment that they plan
to use.

The Positive Deviance Approach

Elements of Improving Quality and Safety in Healthcare

DOI: 10.1017/9781009237130
First published online: August 2022

Ruth Baxter[1] and Rebecca Lawton[1,2]
*[1] Yorkshire Quality and Safety Research Group,
Bradford Institute for Health Research*

[2] School of Psychology, University of Leeds

Author for correspondence: Ruth Baxter, R.M.Baxter@leeds.ac.uk

Abstract: Positive deviance is an asset-based improvement approach. At its core is the belief that solutions to problems already exist within communities, and that identifying, understanding, and sharing these solutions enables improvements at scale. Originating in the field of international public health in the 1960s, positive deviance is now, with some adaptations, seeing growing application in healthcare. This Element presents examples of how positive deviance has been used to support healthcare improvement. The authors draw on an emerging view of safety, known as Safety II, to explain why positive deviance has drawn the interest of researchers and improvers alike. In doing so, they identify a set of fundamental values associated with the positive deviance approach and consider how far they align with current use. Throughout, the authors consider the untapped potential of the approach, reflect on its limitations, and offer insights into the possible challenges of using it in practice. This title is also available as Open Access on Cambridge Core.

Keywords: positive deviance, learning from high performers, Safety II, routinely collected data, qualitative methods

ISBNs: 9781009237116 (PB), 9781009237130 (OC)
ISSNs: 2754-2912 (online), 2754-2904 (print)

Contents

1 Introduction

1.1 What Is Positive Deviance?

Generally speaking, the term 'deviance' can be used to refer to both:

- a behaviour or practice that deviates from the norm and may not be socially acceptable
- an individual or group that is an outlier in terms of their overall performance.

What we describe in this Element uses the second of these meanings. When we refer to positive deviance, we are describing an approach that involves identifying those who demonstrate exceptionally good performance on particular measures (the 'positive deviants') and then trying to understand what allows them to achieve this high level of performance. Their behaviours may differ from the norm, but more importantly they represent behaviours, practices, or systems that facilitate exceptional success.

1.2 The Origins of Positive Deviance and Its Underpinning Assumptions

The term 'positive deviance' was first used in the field of international public health in the 1960s. The approach was fuelled by a backlash against a perceived imperialist, professionalised view of public health interventions, and a move to recognise the knowledge and expertise that already exists within communities. For example, Wray, writing in 1972, describing mothers who were able to keep their children fed in the harshest conditions, proposed that:

> *Such mothers, it would appear, know more than we professionals do. They know how, in that incredible environment, to provide their children with basically adequate diets and to protect them from too frequent infections. Perhaps they can teach us. At the very least, we ought to search out the successful mothers in such circumstances, examine their child care practices, and try to identify what it is they are doing that makes the difference in their children. If we cannot teach these things to other mothers in that environment, perhaps they can.*[1]

The approach is perhaps even more clearly articulated in one of the earliest papers to refer to positive deviance as an alternative approach to studying and improving public health:

> *[T]o identify those families in which a child between age six months and five years falls in the upper 25 per cent in height and weight measurements. These families are labelled as being 'Positive Deviants' from the undernutrition that prevails in the population. They are then studied anthropologically to uncover any practices related to food sources, storage, preparation, consumption, and*

content. The information would be used in designing food supplementation or other nutritional promotion in the population at large on the assumption that the observed 'favourable' practices, although atypical, are feasible and culturally acceptable because they are indigenously rather than extraneously derived.[2]

Most famously, positive deviance was used in the 1990s to improve the nutritional status of children in Vietnam.[3] In this case, an international charity, Save the Children, identified several positively deviant behaviours, including the unusual practice of feeding shrimps from the paddy fields to small children, and other more accepted behaviours, such as hygienic food preparation.[4,5] Through an education programme to help others adopt these practices and behaviours, the organisation saw a 74% reduction in severe malnutrition among children under three years of age. This impact was sustained many years after Save the Children left the communities.[6] Following this, the approach was scaled up to address childhood malnutrition locally and internationally, through a community-based nutrition rehabilitation model combining the positive deviance approach and 'hearth' education sessions.[3] The hearth approach gathers communities around fireplaces or kitchen hearths for education and rehabilitation and to promote the wider adoption of positively deviant behaviours.[7,8] Since then, positive deviance has been used to address various public health issues such as pregnancy outcomes,[9] the care of newborn children,[10] weight control,[11] and female genital mutilation.[12]

Although positive deviance can take different forms, its use in international public health is built on some underpinning assumptions:

- that positive deviants succeed despite facing similar constraints as others
- that solutions to common problems:
  - already exist within communities (in healthcare, these communities are teams, groups, departments, and organisations)
  - can be identified or uncovered by anthropological methods
  - are acceptable, feasible, and sustainable within existing resources because they are already practised by people within the community
- that these features increase the likelihood that the solutions are generalisable to, and can be adopted by, other communities.

1.3 Applying Positive Deviance to Healthcare Improvement

Use of the term 'positive deviance' has increased substantially in recent years, and many different definitions and applications have now emerged.[13] Since the early 2000s, it has expanded into healthcare and has been implemented in diverse ways. Two key frameworks are often used to help operationalise the positive deviance approach: the 4Ds framework and the Bradley et al. framework. These frameworks are explored in more detail next, although it is important to note that some studies offer only poor descriptions of how positive deviance has been implemented in healthcare.[14]

The 4Ds framework (see Figure 1), or variations of it, is most closely aligned to the approach's origins in international public health. It centres around four steps:

- **defining** the problem
- **determining** the presence of positive deviants
- **discovering** the uncommon but successful strategies
- **designing** interventions to allow others to practise these strategies or behaviours.

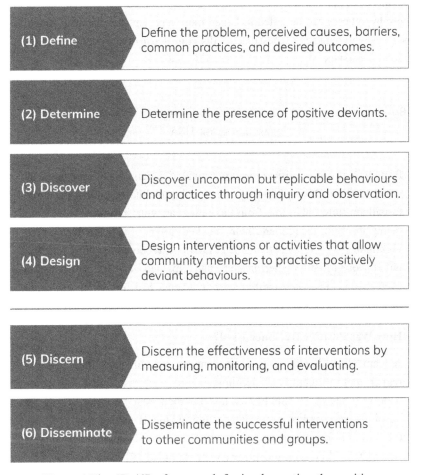

Figure 1 The 4Ds/6Ds framework for implementing the positive deviance approach
Adapted from the Positive Deviance Initiative[15] *and Singhal and Dura.*[16]

Variations of this framework include a fifth[15] and sometimes sixth step,[16] which typically focus on monitoring and evaluating the effectiveness of solutions to support wider dissemination (Figure 1). This framework and its variations have been used across a range of studies, for example to reduce MRSA infections,[16] help smoking cessation among prisoners,[17] and to improve how medical students acquire clinical skills.[18]

Box 1, highlighting research by Bradley et al.,[19] describes one of the most well-known examples of a positive deviance study in healthcare. It led to the development of another four-stage framework (Figure 2) designed to support the positive deviance approach in healthcare organisations specifically. Bradley et al. recommend identifying positive deviants using concrete, routinely collected, and widely endorsed data (stage 1). Qualitative methods should then be used to generate hypotheses about the positively deviant strategies used to succeed (stage 2). These hypotheses can be tested in larger, more representative samples (stage 3), and the newly characterised best practice disseminated to others with the help of key stakeholders (stage 4).

Box 1 IMPROVING DOOR-TO-BALLOON TIMES FOR PATIENTS WITH ACUTE MYOCARDIAL INFARCTION IN THE USA[19-21]

The Problem

Prompt treatment is critical for the survival of patients with acute myocardial infarction. During 2004–05, a national guideline stated that the door-to-balloon time – the time from the patient arriving in hospital to a stent being inserted to reopen their blocked artery – should be within 90 minutes.[22,23] Yet less than 50% of patients received care that met this target. Door-to-balloon performance had remained static for several years, even though other key cardiac care indicators had improved and some hospitals were managing to meet the target.

How Was Positive Deviance Used?

A team of academics, clinical academics, and clinicians used national registry data to identify 35 US hospitals that achieved median door-to-balloon times of 90 minutes or less for their past 50 cases. These 35 hospitals were ranked according to improvements in this measure over the previous four years, and 11 positively deviant hospitals that demonstrated the greatest improvement were sampled. Researchers used in-depth visits (tours and open-ended interviews) at these 11 sites to explore multidisciplinary staff members' perspectives and experiences of improving door-to-balloon times. From their qualitative analysis, the team identified contextual factors (e.g. senior management support, shared goals, physician leaders, and interdisciplinary teams) and specific clinical strategies (e.g. activation of the catheterisation laboratory by emergency medicine physicians instead of cardiologists) that they thought were related to top performance in the positively deviant hospitals.[21]

These qualitative findings were then used to develop a web-based survey, which 365 US hospitals completed. For each hospital, survey data were combined with data on door-to-balloon times, and regression modelling was used to identify six specific clinical strategies that predicted lower door-to-balloon times:[20]

- activation of the catheterisation laboratory by emergency medicine physicians instead of cardiologists
- using a single call to activate the catheterisation team
- activating the catheterisation team while the patient was still en route to hospital
- expecting staff to arrive in the catheterisation laboratory within 20 minutes of being paged
- always having an attending cardiologist on site
- having real-time feedback for staff on door-to-balloon times.

The American College of Cardiology disseminated these findings to other US hospitals via the Door-to-Balloon Alliance – a public campaign supported by 38 professional associations and agencies. Around 70% of hospitals treating acute myocardial infarction signed up to the alliance and, by 2008, the number of patients receiving treatment within 90 minutes had increased by 25%.[19]

The Bradley et al. framework is more data-driven than the 4Ds/6Ds framework, which rarely tests associations between the behaviours and practices identified and the outcomes of interest. It is also more often used at an organisational, regional, or national level (e.g. see studies by Bradley et al., Gabbay et al., and Klaiman et al.[24–28]). Perhaps as a function of this, the framework appears to be predominantly implemented from the top-down, marking a recognisable shift from the original bottom-up applications, where members of the community were integral to all stages of the approach.

Beyond these two frameworks, applications of positive deviance can also broadly be considered to sit on a continuum ranging from those that are 'community driven' to those that are 'externally led'. Positive deviance studies at the community-driven end of the continuum tend to share similarities with those conducted in international public health. Members of the community (i.e. healthcare staff) are typically heavily involved in leading the studies and are central to identifying and creating their own solutions. These studies tend to involve more participatory methods (e.g. discovery and action dialogues or improvisational theatre – see stage 2 of the positive deviance approach in Section 2.2). Though quantitative data can be used, less emphasis is placed on statistically identifying positive deviants and assessing the extent to which their behaviours improve outcomes. Box 2 describes a rigorously conducted community-driven controlled trial in which healthcare staff were integral to identifying positive deviants and how they succeed.[31]

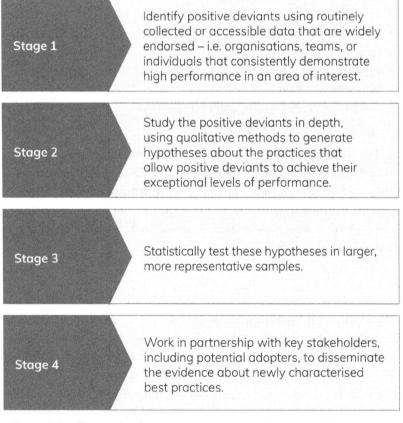

Stage 1 — Identify positive deviants using routinely collected or accessible data that are widely endorsed – i.e. organisations, teams, or individuals that consistently demonstrate high performance in an area of interest.

Stage 2 — Study the positive deviants in depth, using qualitative methods to generate hypotheses about the practices that allow positive deviants to achieve their exceptional levels of performance.

Stage 3 — Statistically test these hypotheses in larger, more representative samples.

Stage 4 — Work in partnership with key stakeholders, including potential adopters, to disseminate the evidence about newly characterised best practices.

Figure 2 Bradley et al.'s four stages to implementing the positive deviance approach in healthcare organisations

Adapted from Bradley et al.,[19] *in accordance with the terms of the Creative Commons licence (http://creativecommons.org/licenses/by/2.0).*

Box 2 USING THE POSITIVE DEVIANCE APPROACH TO ADDRESS HEALTHCARE-ASSOCIATED INFECTIONS

The Problem

Healthcare-associated infections such as Methicillin-resistant *Staphylococcus aureus* (MRSA) are a common cause of ventilator-associated pneumonia, bloodstream infections, and surgical site infections. These infections result in protracted hospital stays and treatment, costing US hospital inpatient services up to $45 billion a year (as estimated in 2007).[29,30] Good hand hygiene effectively prevents healthcare-associated infections, yet behavioural interventions are rarely successful[31] and compliance rates remain relatively low, at around 50%.[29]

How Was Positive Deviance Used?

Marra et al. conducted a controlled trial to improve hand hygiene compliance in two comparable step-down units.[31] After a period of baseline data collection, positive deviance was implemented in one unit, while the other acted as a control. In the intervention unit, nurse managers initially identified positively deviant staff who displayed good hand hygiene compliance. Additional positive deviants were then identified over time. The approach was implemented via twice monthly meetings involving staff who worked across a variety of shifts. Meetings provided opportunities to discuss feelings about hand hygiene, what needed to improve, and examples of good practice. Staff created videos, shared healthcare-associated infection rates, and decided to assess individual performances across shifts to create comparison and competition within the team.

After implementing the positive deviance approach, there was a statistically significant, nearly twofold increase in hand hygiene episodes and a significantly lower infection rate between the intervention and control units.[31] The success of the interventions led to the extension of positive deviance to the control unit after three months of the trial. Throughout, hand hygiene compliance was evaluated using electronic handwashing counters and the incidence of healthcare-associated infections was monitored.

Following this, an observational study explored the sustainability of the positive deviance intervention.[32] For an additional year, staff continued to implement positive deviance on both units and to measure healthcare-associated infections and hand hygiene compliance. Amid concerns that the twice-monthly meetings would become tedious, staff employed motivational techniques (e.g. the parallel thinking process Six Thinking Hats), held interactive sessions to discuss controversial infection control issues, and retained competition among team members. Compared with baseline, each of the two units observed at least a twofold increase in hand hygiene episodes, as well as a significant reduction in the incidence of healthcare-associated infections, suggesting that the improvements gained were sustainable.[32]

By contrast, at the other end of the continuum, externally led applications tend to be much more concerned with accurately identifying positive deviants using quantitative data. This means that these studies are often conducted by outsider experts (e.g. academics, clinical academics, or clinical/national leads), with perhaps less community or frontline participation. These externally led applications may also use rigorous research methods, such as interviews or observations, to understand what is contributing to positive deviance. Broadly, community-driven applications tend to steer more towards applying the 4Ds framework, while externally led applications favour the Bradley et al. framework. However, it is important to note that this is not a dichotomy. Some externally led applications have extensive clinical stakeholder involvement, while some community-driven applications are conducted rigorously and published in peer-reviewed journals.

1.4 What the Approach Is (and What It Is Not)

Traditionally, healthcare has taken a deficit-based, find-and-fix approach to safety management, using methods such as incident reporting and root cause analysis, and producing guidelines and procedures to eliminate the risks identified.[33] This approach to managing safety, now commonly referred to as Safety I, seeks to identify the causes of error and harm to eliminate or contain them. The effectiveness of Safety I has been questioned in recent years,[33,34] resulting in the emergence of the so-called Safety II approach to managing safety.[35,36] Rather than focusing on error and harm, Safety II seeks to understand everyday performance to ensure that as much as possible goes right – that safe care is delivered as frequently as possible under both expected and unexpected conditions.[35] Furthermore, asset-based approaches, such as Learning from Excellence[37] and appreciative inquiry,[38] are increasingly used to improve both the quality and safety of care. Safety II and asset-based approaches share elements in common with positive deviance: they focus on identifying and learning from what goes right rather than being dominated by what has gone wrong and, broadly speaking, they seek to understand 'work as done' rather than 'work as imagined'.

The positive deviance approach is distinctive, however (Table 1). For example, Safety II seeks to generate learning from everyday performance,

Table 1 Key differences between Safety I, Safety II, and the positive deviance approach

	Safety I	Safety II	Positive deviance
Underpinning premise	To ensure that as few things as possible go wrong. Focus on negative outliers.	To ensure that as many things as possible go right. Focus on everyday performance.	To learn from those who demonstrate exceptional performance on outcomes of interest. Focus on positive outliers.
Safety management principle	Reactive – respond when something happens or risk is deemed unacceptable.	Proactive – continually try to anticipate developments and events.	Either reactive or proactive – learn from those who overcome specific problems *or* learn from those who achieve excellence.
View of human factors	Humans are predominantly seen as a liability or hazard. They are a problem to be fixed.	Humans are seen as a resource for system flexibility and resilience. They provide flexible solutions to potential problems.	Humans are seen as a source of exceptional performance – they have developed solutions to overcome problems as individuals or within groups.
Investigations	Accidents are caused by failures and malfunctions. The purpose of an investigation is to identify the causes.	Things go wrong for the same reasons that they go right. The purpose of an investigation is to understand how care usually goes right, as a basis for explaining how care occasionally goes wrong.	Exceptional performance is caused by positively deviant behaviours. The purpose of an investigation is to identify these behaviours and learn from them.

Adapted from Hollnagel et al.[35]

rather than focusing on extreme performance outliers.[35,36] Acknowledging the complexity of healthcare, Safety II assumes that good and bad outcomes occur in the same way and that safe care is created by people constantly adapting and adjusting to the variable conditions and situations that they face.[35,36] By contrast, positive deviance takes a more linear approach assuming that it is possible to identify and then spread the causes of exceptional performance – the behaviours or processes that reliably lead to exceptional outcomes. Although positive deviance shifts our gaze to the opposite end of the performance spectrum, it could, in essence, be considered akin to a Safety I approach, albeit one that focuses on finding and fixing (i.e. spreading) the causes of sustained positive performances rather than one-off negative incidents or events.

Similar distinctions can be drawn between positive deviance and approaches such as Learning from Excellence and appreciative inquiry. Learning from Excellence aims to improve quality of care and staff morale through peer-reported episodes of success, which are shared and, in some instances, discussed or analysed in more depth to generate learning.[39] Despite its name, Learning from Excellence typically focuses on discrete episodes of *everyday* success that arise through workarounds, improvisations, and the generosity of staff.[40] By contrast, positive deviance focuses on exceptional performance outliers who typically sustain exceptional performance over time.

Appreciative inquiry is a participatory approach that generates organisational change by reframing problems, building on positive ideas, and fostering learning.[38,41] Although appreciative inquiry is used in some applications of positive deviance to uncover success (particularly those that are community-driven or conducted in international public health), it does not specifically seek to learn from those who demonstrate exceptional performance.[42]

2 The Positive Deviance Approach in Action

Positive deviance has been applied to healthcare improvement at different levels of the system and to address a variety of different problems. This section is structured around Bradley et al.'s framework, as it is thus far the only one that has been designed specifically for healthcare settings.[19] We present cases that exemplify each stage, while also drawing on examples of community-driven applications. Cases are used to highlight some of the challenges and the opportunities of using the positive deviance approach.

2.1 Stage 1: Identifying Positive Deviants

Identifying positive deviants is fundamental to the positive deviance approach, regardless of which framework is followed. Bradley et al. suggest using routinely collected, accessible data to do so.[19] Three major challenges must be overcome at this stage of the approach: measurement, which is notoriously difficult in healthcare; how to analyse the available data to identify exceptional performers; and making like-for-like comparisons to identify true positive deviants.

2.1.1 Measurement in Healthcare Is Notoriously Difficult

The quality and safety of patient care is measured via outcomes and processes. Outcomes relate to observed measures of morbidity and mortality and so are of greatest interest to patients, clinicians, improvers, and policy-makers. However, process measures, which measure performance based on adherence to established clinical standards, are often more sensitive to differences in the quality of care.[43] When looking to apply the positive deviance approach to some improvement problems, routinely collected or accessible outcome data simply do not exist.[44–46] Where outcome data do exist, they may not be useful. This may be because clinical outcome data represent a measure that is too blunt (e.g. 'all' rather than 'avoidable' readmissions) or distal (e.g. mortality). In these situations, process measures may provide a more accurate measure.[43,47] For example, if assessing the success of a public health campaign, bowel cancer screening rates could be measured rather than bowel cancer cases.

Furthermore, the expression 'garbage in, garbage out' is highly relevant to data issues in applications of positive deviance. Through our own work[48] – to explore what routinely available data are available to compare the safety performance of wards, units, and services – we identified some of the pitfalls. They include problems with the measures used to collect data, such as a mandatory staff survey question that asks: 'When errors, near misses or incidents are reported, my organisation takes action to ensure that they do not happen again.' At first sight, this item seems reasonable. But, if the organisation's action is to discipline everyone who makes a mistake, a positive value on this item does not necessarily indicate an organisation that demonstrates safety. Likewise, if reported incidents are used to measure safety, the motivations to report are likely to skew the outcome. People may not report incidents because they are fearful, while others might report incidents, including near misses, in an attempt to get something done about a problem they experience regularly (e.g. short-staffing). Self-reported data are subject to many influences that can make them unreliable for comparing organisations.

To be useful, data also need to be accessible. Data are not always publicly available or collected in a standardised way (e.g. clinical coding can vary across organisations), making it difficult to compare performances across organisations. Furthermore, data may not be available at a level that is relevant to the aims of the study. For example, hospital readmission data are published at speciality level, making it difficult to explore how ward teams achieve exceptionally safe hospital discharges. Though some data are available at team or individual level (e.g. for surgical outcomes[49] and national clinical audits[50]), it is often sparse, unavailable, or very difficult or costly to obtain.

2.1.2 How to Analyse the Available Data to Identify Exceptional Performers

Many applications of positive deviance rank performance data and identify positive deviants as those who perform best.[14] However, rankings (e.g. in league tables) may not actually identify the best and worst performers.[51–53] It is also important to consider the time frame over which positive deviants demonstrate exceptional performance. Some studies identify and learn from one-off successes,[18] while in others positive deviants must sustain their performance over a period of time.[48,54] Since a one-off outlying status may not be a reliable indicator of success, it may be preferable to learn from those who have demonstrated excellence over a longer period of time.

A variety of sophisticated statistical techniques can be used to identify high performers, but statistical process control methods are increasingly promoted as an accessible way of measuring variation within healthcare.[47,55,56] These methods combine statistical rigour with the ability to sensitively measure performance variation – they distinguish between variation that is to be expected (noise) and variation that may have an assignable cause (e.g. variation that may result from the presence of positive or negative deviants). The methods are sensitive to small sample sizes, can facilitate temporal analysis, and the visual rather than tabular presentation of data makes it easier to identify performance outliers.[57] For more information, see the Element on statistical process control.[58]

2.1.3 Making Like-for-Like Comparisons to Identify True Positive Deviants

The third challenge relates to an underpinning assumption of the approach – that positive deviants succeed despite facing similar constraints as others. This is important, because, for example, some apparent high performers may succeed simply because they care for a less complex or acute patient population, or because the service is better funded. It is important that study samples are carefully selected to account, control for, or minimise confounding variables so that, as far as possible, like-for-like comparisons are made. Nevertheless, accurate case-mix adjustments are often extremely difficult and, depending on how they are made, different high and low performers may be identified. Some confounders will also always remain unmeasured and thus unaccounted for within the adjustments. For a more detailed discussion of this, see Lilford et al.[43]

2.1.4 Could a Non-Data-Driven Method Be a Solution?

If the positive deviance approach is to be distinguished from other asset-based improvement approaches, based on its premise of learning from exceptional performers, then positive deviants should represent an outlying population. To overcome the challenges above, several studies have identified positive deviants in non-data-driven ways, for example by selecting award nominees.[59,60] Marra et al.[31,32,61] identified positive deviants using tacit knowledge rather than data (see Box 2 for an overview of the study). Initially, nurse managers identified healthcare workers who they considered to be positively deviant and, over time, these individuals identified other positive deviants within their team. Positive deviants displayed good hand hygiene compliance, had a desire to change and develop ideas, and stimulated compliance across the team.[31] Alternatively, some projects, predominantly those that are community-driven, do not identify positively deviant individuals or teams. Instead, discovery and action dialogues (see stage 2 in Section 2.2) are used to define and generate ownership of problems and to identify uncommon behaviours or practices. When positive deviants are identified in non-data-driven ways, it is not known whether they truly display *exceptional* performance. However, despite this, Marra et al. were able to demonstrate significant improvements in hand hygiene compliance and associated outcomes.[31,32,61]

2.2 Stage 2: Generating Hypotheses about How Positive Deviants Succeed

In this stage, qualitative methods are used to generate hypotheses about the positively deviant strategies that facilitate exceptional performance.[19] In our own work, we have explored how positively deviant older people's medical ward teams deliver exceptionally safe patient care, as measured by the UK's National Health Service (NHS) Safety Thermometer data – a routinely collected measure of four commonly occurring harms.[54,62,63] We conducted multidisciplinary focus groups and informal observations on four positively deviant and four above-average comparator wards to gather a wide range of perspectives and generate discussion about how teams successfully deliver safe patient care. We also made brief field notes following each focus group to capture factors such as team dynamics. In total, 14 positively deviant characteristics were identified, such as knowing one another well, working together, having integrated allied health professionals, and team stability. These characteristics were either present only on the positively deviant wards or enacted in a substantially different way on the positively deviant wards compared with the comparators.[63]

This study illustrates some important considerations for undertaking stage 2 of the positive deviance approach: what lens should be applied and should a framework be used to guide data collection; do teams have the skills and capacity required; how might sampling and comparators influence the hypotheses generated; and are there other ways to create opportunities for discussion to generate learning?

2.2.1 Consider What Lens to Apply to Qualitative Data Collection

Many studies focus on specific processes and outcomes of care, such as providing weight loss advice[64] or anticoagulation control.[65] Bounding the scope of studies may make it more feasible to generate an in-depth nuanced understanding of the behaviours or processes that facilitate success, particularly if time and resources are limited. However, in doing so, it is still important to apply a broad lens so as to explicate the wider contextual influences (e.g. policies, leadership, and culture) that facilitate success and to illuminate any unintended consequences (positive or negative) that may arise from the positively deviant strategies. If trying to improve narrow processes or outcomes of care, it is important to think broadly about the factors that may influence exceptional performance and direct the qualitative gaze appropriately.

Alternatively, studies may want to explore how positive deviants succeed on broad outcomes of care to deliver high-quality or safe care in the round. For example, rather than focusing on specific harms (e.g. falls or pressure ulcers), our study on medical wards for older people explored how teams deliver exceptionally safe care across a range of measures.[63] By looking at those who succeed across a bigger picture, it may be possible to uncover latent factors that facilitate their success – the upstream, system-level factors that are more difficult to observe, such as staffing and skill mix, leadership style, culture, and physical environment. In doing so, it may be possible to target these latent factors to generate improvement across a range of outcomes.

2.2.2 Consider Using a Framework to Guide the Collection of Qualitative Data

Regardless of which lens is taken, qualitative data collection and analysis in positive deviance studies may benefit from using a theoretical framework to help ensure that factors underpinning exceptional performance are comprehensively assessed.[14,66,67] For example, Rose et al. structured their qualitative enquiry in anticoagulation clinics around nine key domains that were considered essential to establishing and maintaining a high-quality anticoagulation control.[65] For patient safety research, the Yorkshire Contributory Factors Framework[68] or the Manchester Patient Safety Framework[69] might be useful.

Beyond safety, researchers or improvers could use frameworks such as the COM-B behaviour change wheel[70] or the PARIHS (Promoting Action on Research Implementation in Health Services) framework.[71] Nonetheless, care must also be taken. Positive deviance is inherently an inductive (i.e. emergent) approach.[11] If applied rigidly, the use of a theory or framework might bias the data generated and blind the observer to those unusual, perhaps deviant practices or factors that might have been identified inductively or that fall outside the scope of the particular theory or framework used.

2.2.3 Tailor the Method to the Skills and Capacity of the Teams Involved

In choosing a method to generate hypotheses about how success is achieved, those conducting a positive deviance study should consider the skills and capacity within their teams. Particularly among externally led applications of positive deviance, a common approach to generate hypotheses about success has been to use ethnographic methods such as extensive observations and formal or informal interviews. These methods facilitate a robust in-depth inquiry and may be well suited to uncovering the beliefs, values, and assumptions that underpin success on broad outcomes of care. For example, Liberati et al.[72] conducted an ethnography consisting of approximately 143 hours of observation, semi-structured interviews, and focus groups to explore how a maternity unit in England achieved and sustained exceptional safety outcomes.

Yet these methods are rarely accessible to frontline clinicians and improvement organisations (e.g. national audit teams, clinical commissioning groups) that may lack the capability and capacity required to conduct them. If positive deviance is to be used for healthcare improvement, as distinct from research, it may be necessary to challenge one of the underpinning assumptions of positive deviance: that success should be uncovered anthropologically. Our study on older people's medical wards[63] tested pragmatic methods that were more (although not completely) accessible to an improvement community. We found that relationships across the multidisciplinary teams enabled people to know one another socially, as well as understand and value each other's roles. The teams worked to extremely high standards and expectations, and staff could raise safety concerns or ask for emotional and technical help when needed.

These findings share similarities with those produced by the more extended investigations undertaken by Liberati et al.[72] and so, given this, it may be possible to develop a method that is both feasible within an improvement context and sufficient for generating robust hypotheses about how positive deviants succeed. Future research could usefully explore the extent to which different methods can generate robust hypotheses at stage 2, and what the resource implications of these different methods are.

2.2.4 Consider How Sampling and Comparators May Influence the Hypotheses that Are Generated

Having a comparator is a useful addition to a positive deviance study, not least because it is important to understand how positive deviants differ from the rest of a population. Many positive deviance studies do not sample comparators during stage 2 and, where they do, they tend to be negative deviants – the worst performers in a population.[14] The stark comparison provided by sampling positive and negative deviants may make it easier to identify very obvious differences between the two groups. However, this comparison does not necessarily help identify behaviours and strategies that distinguish positive deviants from those in a population who simply perform well – those with average performances. Sampling comparators that demonstrate good or average performances may help uncover how positive deviants differ from the majority of a population in order to achieve truly exceptional performance.

It is also important to consider how many positive deviants and comparators to sample. Sampling multiple positive deviants and comparators (e.g. Baxter et al.[63] and Curry et al.[73]) may lead to more generalisable hypotheses, whereas sampling a single positive deviant (e.g. Liberati et al.[72] and Hughes et al.[74]) may help generate an in-depth picture of exceptional performance within that particular context.

2.2.5 Create Opportunities for Discussion to Generate Learning

Many positive deviance studies do not necessarily use rigorous research methods to uncover positively deviant strategies. Particularly when following the 4Ds framework, some, as we noted above, use discovery and action dialogues. For these dialogues, interested people are brought together for facilitated discussions to uncover positively deviant practices (and positive deviants in some cases), to generate new solutions for improvement, and to identify ways of overcoming existing barriers.[75] For example, in trying to reduce bloodstream infections, Lindberg et al.[76] used discovery and action dialogues to discuss infection causes, strategies and barriers to prevent infection, whether certain people frequently overcame these barriers, other improvement ideas, and how these ideas might be initiated. Other studies use improvisational theatre in which short dramas and scenarios are acted out, providing frontline staff with a social, sensory, and collaborative way to learn and discover together.[77]

2.3 Stage 3: Testing Hypotheses in Larger Samples

In stage 3, the hypotheses generated during stage 2 can be tested in larger, more representative samples to explore their associations with improved outcomes.[19] Few publications explicitly report this stage of the framework; we use Bradley et al.'s original research[20] to exemplify this stage.

2.3.1 Using a Survey to Test the Hypotheses

Box 1 outlines Bradley et al.'s use of national registry data to identify 11 positively deviant US hospitals that had consistently achieved and shown improvements in the 90-minute door-to-balloon time target. After identifying several processes and organisational contextual factors that were thought to facilitate exceptional performance,[21] the researchers conducted stage 3 by creating a web-based survey to explore the extent to which hospitals within the wider community implemented the processes that had been identified.[20] The survey addressed 28 key hospital strategies that could be objectively and reliably measured using close-ended, multiple choice questions (e.g. the process for activating the catheterisation team). It was piloted for clarity and comprehensiveness, and then distributed to 500 hospitals across the USA.

Hierarchical generalised linear modelling was used to identify six hospital strategies that were associated with significantly faster door-to-balloon times (e.g. the emergency department activating the catheterisation laboratory while the patient is en route to hospital, and always having an attending cardiologist on site). Some of these associations were particularly strong and were estimated to save 10–15 minutes. Hospitals with faster door-to-balloon times had implemented more of the effective strategies.

2.3.2 How Useful Is Stage 3?

Bradley et al.'s study[20] highlights the benefits of conducting stage 3 of the positive deviance approach. By testing hypotheses in larger, more representative samples, they demonstrated which strategies were associated with improved outcomes and dismissed those that were not, allowing them to focus on the most important strategies. Stage 3 complements an evidence-based approach to medicine and enables resources to be directed in ways that are most likely to generate improvement. Quantitative evidence, such as this, can also provide a powerful motivator for change by convincing others that strategies are worth adopting.[78]

Nonetheless, there are various challenges to conducting stage 3. First, cross-sectional surveys only demonstrate correlation – not causation – and so implementing strategies may not improve outcomes. Furthermore, the direction of the relationship between strategies and outcomes is not always clear. In some cases, exceptional performance may lead to the positively deviant factors observed, rather than the other way round; for example, exceptional performance may generate high levels of job satisfaction within positively deviant teams.[63]

Second, positively deviant strategies are not always amenable to measurement. Routinely collected data are rarely available to adequately assess the hypotheses that are generated through stage 2. It can be difficult to simplify positively deviant strategies into discrete survey items, and to generate valid and reliable questions that sufficiently measure the hypotheses. Furthermore, asking people to rate themselves, their teams, or their organisations presents its own challenges. Survey questions are open to interpretation, especially if they have not been validated. These problems are most pertinent if the survey is assessing contextual or cultural factors, rather than whether specific processes, policies, or procedures are in place. In this case, the contribution of latent factors (e.g. leadership, psychological safety) in facilitating success may be downplayed.

Some community-driven applications of positive deviance collect data to continually monitor performance throughout the life cycle of improvement. This allows improvers to observe the effects of positive deviance strategies on performance,[79] although it is not always clear from the published research articles which changes in practice actually produced any improvements in performance (e.g. when bundles of interventions are implemented). In addition to measuring processes and outcomes, many community-driven applications use social network analysis to measure the impact of positive deviance. This does not provide a measure of the effectiveness of specific positively deviant practices, but can provide an indicator of culture change, which often accompanies the ability to overcome 'wicked issues': challenges that are complex and multifaceted, and are therefore beyond the ability of any one organisation to handle in isolation.[76,79,80]

Given the difficulties of measurement and testing associations between positively deviant strategies and outcomes – particularly when these strategies represent latent or upstream factors (e.g. culture and leadership) rather than more concrete processes or strategies – further critical appraisal of the worth of this stage of the framework is needed. While it is important to develop improvement strategies and processes based on rigorous evidence, qualitative evidence may be sufficient when identifying cultural factors (e.g. trusting relationships, people who know one another) that serve to underpin good outcomes.

2.4 Stage 4: Disseminating Positively Deviant Strategies to Others

In stage 4, positively deviant strategies are disseminated to others in the wider population with the help of key stakeholders.[19] There are very few published examples of this stage. One possible explanation is that articles simply do not refer to a positive deviance framework and so dissemination activities cannot be linked to applications of the approach, or it may represent a time lag between completing and publishing this final stage. Another interpretation is that the positive deviance studies may have failed to produce generalised improvement.

2.4.1 Different Approaches to Dissemination

Due to the dearth of literature on this stage, we refer again to the work of Bradley et al., who disseminated their positively deviant strategies with the support of a group of highly influential organisations.[81] The American College of Cardiology, in partnership with the American Heart Association and 37 other organisations, implemented a well-coordinated and highly promoted national campaign called the Door-to-Balloon Alliance. When healthcare organisations signed up to the alliance, they committed to treat at least 75% of patients within the 90-minute window, and benefitted from a toolkit and change programme based on the positive deviance evidence, individually tailored actions plans, educational initiatives (e.g. workshops, seminars, and an online community), and regional champions to help motivate and facilitate change. Contextually the alliance was set up at a time when national reporting and financial incentives were also being implemented. Evaluation of the alliance showed significant three-year improvements in door-to-balloon times, whereby 25% more patients received treatment within the 90-minute window than before.[19]

By contrast, Sreeramoju et al.[82] took a different approach to spread practices to reduce healthcare-associated infections. Researchers implemented a positive deviance intervention on three randomly selected wards. They conducted interviews and focus groups, collected data via graffiti boards and drop boxes, and identified 12 positively deviant individuals. To disseminate their findings and generate improvement (equivalent to stage 4), the positive deviants, along with the ward managers, infection preventionists, and a research team member, created an action planning group to help spread and implement some of the ideas. The group used the data that had been gathered to sort, prioritise, implement, and evaluate the improvement ideas that had been generated, often through plan-do-study-act (PDSA) cycles. Importantly, it was the healthcare staff, rather than the researchers, who owned these plans. Compared with three randomly selected control wards, the positive deviance intervention significantly impacted a trend in patient safety culture (prevented a decline), although no differences were found in social network maps or healthcare-associated infections.

2.4.2 Top-Down versus Bottom-Up Dissemination

These two examples highlight the different ways in which positively deviant strategies can be disseminated. Bradley et al.[19,81] took a top-down approach – national organisations created the alliance. By contrast, Sreeramoju et al.'s approach[82] was more bottom-up – although external researchers supported the earlier qualitative work, findings were acted upon and improvement projects were owned by members of the ward teams. There is limited evidence to say which approach is the most effective, and in what circumstances.

Top-down approaches may be better suited to organisation and system-level applications of positive deviance, where influence is required to instigate change at a regional or national level. A bottom-up approach to dissemination is more aligned with the original international public health and community-driven applications of positive deviance. They may suit individual or team level applications, where it is easier to promote the meaningful community involvement. A bottom-up approach may also be better suited to disseminating positively deviant strategies that are less concrete and tangible (e.g. cultural factors), as bringing communities together may enable them to gather a more nuanced understanding of how success is achieved, making it more likely that they will adopt the strategies and appreciate the relevance to their own context. When planning positive deviance studies, greater attention should be given to the role of communities (e.g. staff and patients) and how they can be effectively involved in the approach without it becoming too burdensome.

2.4.3 How Closely Should Others Replicate the Strategies?

A further unanswered question relating to stage 4 is whether other individuals, teams, organisations, and so on should seek to replicate and mimic positively deviant strategies, or instead adopt only their underlying premise. The importance of context in quality improvement is well recognised.[83] Many successful interventions have failed to scale: they do not achieve the same impacts in wards or organisations that were not involved in the original improvement project (e.g. Bion et al.[84] and Dixon-Woods et al.[85]). Again, the extent to which positively deviant strategies should be mimicked or adapted (and in what ways) may depend on whether it is a procedural or cultural strategy that is being disseminated. In either situation though, it is important that the qualitative inquiries (stage 2) explore not just *what* positively deviants do to succeed, but also *how* they achieve these things, and the contextual factors that support or hinder them.

To summarise the four stages in this section, Table 2 outlines some of the key barriers to implementing the positive deviance approach and offers potential strategies to mitigate them.

3 Critiques of the Positive Deviance Approach

The use of positive deviance as an improvement approach in healthcare is relatively new, with much of the research published in the past 10–15 years. It is also fair to say that most positive deviance studies in the field are reported in a largely uncritical way. As we have described elsewhere,[14] limitations include limited detail on how positively deviant individuals or teams were identified, under-use of comparisons and controls, and absent or poorly reported involvement of staff and patients. Despite the lack of critical reflection in the studies themselves, some opinion and thought pieces that espouse the value of positive deviance do acknowledge its limitations and the difficulties of applying it at scale.[19,67,90] Here we describe the key issues to consider before choosing to adopt a positive deviance approach.

3.1 Robust Discoveries Require Robust Data

When embarking on a positive deviance project, it is vital that someone in the team understands data, and that all involved are encouraged to adopt a critical stance on the data, identifying only those measures that are reliable, valid, and meet a set of previously agreed criteria. These problems with poor quality data are not unique to positive deviance.[46] Many improvement approaches (e.g. see the Element on audit, feedback, and behaviour change[91]) rely on data either to drive the improvement or to evaluate its impact. Indeed, these same data are used to identify, and take action against, negative deviants.

Given the challenges of identifying positive deviants accurately, it is important to consider the extent to which we should prevent the perfect from being the enemy of the good. If we can improve by learning from those who perform well, rather than from those who perform exceptionally well, perhaps a more pragmatic approach should be embraced. It could be argued that the risk of promoting a practice that is not definitively associated with the highest performing teams or services may be lower than reconfiguring or closing down a service that has been identified to be a negative deviant.

Table 2 Barriers to implementing the positive deviance approach (as designed by Bradley et al.[19]) and potential strategies for mitigation

Barrier	Potential mitigation
Routinely collected data are not available at the level required (e.g. hospital or individual level) to assess the outcome that I am interested in.	• Consider an alternative implementation approach. • Or, if you have the resources, collect your own data (see Kim et al.[86] and Awofeso et al.[17] as examples). • Or consider alternative non-data-driven methods for identifying excellence. Ask the community.

I don't have much confidence in the quality of the data.	• Consider an alternative improvement approach.
	• Or, if possible, increase confidence by:
	  ○ using data recorded over multiple time points
	  ○ using multiple sources of data that measure the same thing, and look for similar patterns across different sources
	  ○ identifying a site as a positive deviant only when it has demonstrated consistently high performance, sustained improvement, and/or high performance across multiple measures.
	• Or consider a non-data-driven method to identify positive deviants (e.g. select award winners or use tacit knowledge uncovered through discovery and action dialogues).

I don't have the specialist skills that are required to analyse the data.	Although skills in statistical process control were rare a few years ago, now many data managers in healthcare and research organisations have these skills. Ask for help.

I am concerned that the organisation(s), units, or people identified as positive deviants might not be.

With good data and analyses, and by controlling for factors that are known to lead to greater success (e.g. higher amounts of funding, a younger patient population, fewer comorbidities), you can largely avoid this risk. However, it is important to involve the community you are interested in. For example, you might identify five maternity units as positive deviants, but then the doctors and midwives in your community tell you that site four (of these five) is a specialist centre, with higher levels of funding that attracts all of the best junior doctors. Formally then, this site does not succeed despite facing similar constraints as others. It is useful to know this and to understand what resources impact performance, but it should not be included as a positively deviant site for further investigation.

I am worried that excellence might not actually be excellence (related to the barrier above).

This is a trap that everyone working in this field needs to be aware of and is why working with the community is so important. Say, for example, you were conducting a study that focuses on injury during restraint in mental health settings. You identify three sites where injury from restraint is much lower. The problem here is a lack of denominator (i.e. the number of restraints), but more worrying is that without assessing the use of anti-psychotics you do not know whether lack of injury is simply a function of fewer restraints due to over-medication. So, always be aware of these balancing measures in your analysis.

I don't have a theory to frame the qualitative work.

The use of a theoretical framework or programme theory should be given due consideration. However, it is important that you are prepared for the unexpected. Positive deviance is an inductive not a deductive process – rather than rigidly applying an existing theory or framework, new data and observations should be gathered with as few preconceptions as possible.

Table 2 (cont.)

Barrier	Potential mitigation
	What is more important is that you understand the field of practice and work with the community to help you generate your own model. This will very much depend on your analytical lens – is it on a very specific outcome (e.g. injury during restraint in mental health settings), or is it on a broad outcome (e.g. patient experience)? The framework you use will differ accordingly. As a minimum, try to ensure that your lens is on both the practices themselves and the context in which they are supported.
I don't know which qualitative method to use.	Your choice of method will depend on your question and the topic of your study. Interviews may be appropriate if focusing on positively deviant individuals or very simple/concrete processes of care. Focus groups and observations may be more useful for complex or broader issues. Particularly for improvement rather than research studies, the choice of method may also be influenced by pragmatics (e.g. skill mix, resources, and time).
	It is worth noting that people are not always very good at telling you what they are doing to achieve success, so if you can build in an ethnographic method (e.g. observation) for data collection, then this is likely to be more productive. If you are limited by time and resources, focus groups can be very useful, particularly if you are interested in team dynamics.
I am not sure how to test the hypotheses that I have generated about factors leading to success.	As part of a Safety I approach to safety management, it is rarely possible to test hypotheses about factors leading to failure before implementing interventions based on these ideas, so, at one level, you could argue that stage 3 is not essential. There is also little evidence about the importance of this stage or the rigour with which it can be conducted. In some cases, it is very simple to conduct,

for example, if you have routinely collected data (e.g. audits) that assess outcomes relating to the specific hypotheses you have generated. However, this is not always possible. As a minimum, we recommend checking the face validity of the hypotheses with members of the population that you are working with – do clinicians and/or patients think the hypotheses are likely to be associated with improved outcomes?

Implementing or spreading the ideas is difficult.	For guidance, see the Elements on collaboration-based approaches,[87] making culture change happen,[88] and approaches to spread, scale-up, and sustainability.[89] There is no magic bullet, sadly!
	Members of the community you have worked with to deliver the project can be very powerful advocates for the findings – try and involve them when disseminating positively deviant strategies. In our research,[63,74] staff have engaged positively with an approach that asks them to reflect success and solutions rather than failure and problems.
	Community members are also likely to have access to professional groups and national bodies, as well as informal and local networks that can support implementation. You can evidence that the positively deviant strategies produce excellent outcomes, and you know that they have worked elsewhere in similar contexts – capitalise on this when capturing the hearts and minds of those you are disseminating to.

We use 'community' to refer to the group of people who deliver (and receive) the care under investigation, and staff who deliver care, have patient contact, or administer the process of patient care.

Nonetheless, caution should be applied: focusing on the wrong positive deviants may lead to learning that is actually counterproductive for improvement.

3.2 Using Positive Deviance in Healthcare Is Unlikely to Uncover Surprises

Using positive deviance in healthcare organisations in high-income countries is very different from its origins in international public health. The solutions identified in studies of healthcare are rarely exceptionally *deviant*. They are not, typically, like shrimps in the paddy fields, the unusual practices so often associated with early positive deviance work in Vietnam.[4,5] Solutions identified in positively deviant healthcare teams and organisations are often things that are acceptable to others; they may be commonly known or evidence based, but perhaps just not uniformly adopted. For example, using alcohol gel in addition to soap and water rather than relying on just one or the other when ensuring hand hygiene prior to central line insertion.[92] Alternatively, the hypotheses generated by qualitatively studying positive deviants in depth (stage 2 of the Bradley et al. framework) may be structural or cultural. They might be about psychological safety and trust in multidisciplinary teams, common goals, and transformational leadership. In fact, what these findings might suggest, and it is difficult with the current evidence to deny, is that positive deviance in healthcare may be synonymous with the ability to identify good practice and the contexts that facilitate their achievement.

3.3 The Positive Deviance Approach Must Account for the Complexity of the Healthcare System

Healthcare organisations are complex[93] and, as such, systems often act in unpredictable ways to produce emergent outcomes. International public health and some of the more community-driven positive deviance studies have been cognisant of this complexity. They have, for example, used participatory methods that engage frontline staff, foster relationships/networks, encourage diverse participation and perspectives, and empower staff to make decisions (see Lindberg and Schneider[94] for further discussion). Through this, the positive deviance approach is able to influence the parameters that shape self-organisation in complex adaptive systems – the natural and local emergence of order, innovation, and progress. Namely, it improves information flow, enhances the number and quality of connections, includes diverse perspectives, and shifts power differentials.[94] However, it might be argued that positive deviance, particularly as conceptualised in Bradley et al.'s framework or by externally led applications, fails to recognise this complexity.

Limited community involvement risks a loss of engagement, connections, diversity, and empowerment, instead reducing the approach to simply *finding* specific solutions and spreading these to others to *fix* problems – a somewhat reductionist and linear approach to generating improvement. For positive deviance, key qualities are its asset-based character and its commitment to learning from the bottom up. It is important, then, that the underpinning principle that communities themselves hold the expertise and skill is not lost in a hierarchical healthcare system where policies, targets, and regulation are externally driven.

3.4 Applications Need to Explore the Mechanisms of Change

At the beginning of this Element, we outlined a set of underlying assumptions of positive deviance: solutions exist within communities; positive deviants succeed despite facing similar constraints; and this tacit knowledge can be generalised to others. In addition, Marsh et al. have proposed that the approach facilitates three important mechanisms of change:[95] *social mobilisation,* whereby communities are motivated to engage with the approach; *information gathering*, to identify behaviours that facilitate good outcomes; and *behaviour change,* whereby the wider community adopts these new behaviours. The way that positive deviance has been operationalised in healthcare, a sector where quantitative evidence is central to decision-making, may mean that the mechanisms of social mobilisation and behaviour change have been lost in translation. For example, social mobilisation (bottom-up community involvement) has a central role in many of the typically community-driven studies, but, in the externally led studies, particularly at organisational level, this aspect is typically missing almost completely. If improvers are to stay true to the origins of positive deviance, then it is important that studies clearly align with the underlying assumption of actively involving positive deviants in identifying solutions and spreading them to others. Without social mobilisation, behaviour change becomes something that has to be done at the end of the project to ensure the spread of practices, rather than being an integral part of the process of conducting positive deviance. As such, applications of positive deviance that lack community involvement may face the same implementation challenges, including behaviour change, of any other quality improvement approach.

3.5 There Is a Lot We Do Not Yet Know about Positive Deviance

The use of positive deviance in healthcare is very much in its infancy, meaning there are many questions about its use and effectiveness still to be answered.

Much more needs to be understood about how positive deviance works and what the mechanisms of action are. For example, given our aforementioned comments, how critical are social mobilisation, information gathering, and behaviour change? In what ways is positive deviance distinctive or advantageous compared with other improvement approaches? For example, a comparative study that explores the processes and outcomes of audit and feedback versus, or perhaps combined with, positive deviance is one possible avenue for further research.

Future research also needs to test different ways of conducting the qualitative stage of positive deviance. It is important to identify what level of effort is sufficient for generating reliable hypotheses about the factors underpinning excellence. This is even more critical if these hypotheses will not be tested in larger samples before implementation. To what extent should we learn from those who truly outperform? What is the most appropriate comparator group? How important is the wider testing of hypotheses? What do we spread – specific practices, or contextual and relational factors, or both?

One other important but unanswered question is the extent to which the learning from one context can be applied to another. This applies both to specific practices and processes as well as to the structural and cultural features of organisations. In our work in two very different settings (elective hip and knee surgery[74] and older people's care[54,62,63]) we have found that while some of our findings were similar in both settings (strong multidisciplinary teams and psychological safety), other factors were entirely different, reflecting the nature of these two services. In the more predictable elective service, reliability and standardisation of process were key, whereas in the more unpredictable older people's service, personalisation and adaptability were critical. Based on these and other findings, we would hypothesise that there will be some fundamental and transferable learning about cultural and structural factors that facilitate excellence across settings and that the growing evidence base will allow, through systematic review, identification of these. But, in addition, there will be other factors (practices, processes, and ways of working) that are not generalisable beyond the service, specialty, or client group.

4 Conclusions

Positive deviance offers a set of core ideas: expertise being held within communities, the importance of learning from communities that succeed, and mobilising communities to spread the learning. Positive deviance resonates with the changing landscape of quality and safety research and improvement, particularly in its growing attempt to understand 'work as done' rather than 'work as imagined' – a distinction that is at the fore of Safety II thinking. Adopting positive deviance enables learning from the experts doing the work rather than those who commission or regulate the work. This is attractive in conditions where the strain on healthcare resources is high and approaches to improvement based on what is imagined are likely to be increasingly removed from the reality of what is achievable.

Despite its challenges, positive deviance remains promising, particularly as the availability of good quality and cross-sector data grow. As with any relatively new approach, however, many questions remain to be answered about its optimal use and the extent to which findings in one domain are generalisable to another. We must also be prepared to be more critical in applying and evaluating this approach than we have been to date. Finally, it will be important to reflect on the way that positive deviance is being applied in healthcare, with its strong focus on rigorous research methods and data. This may mean losing some of the espoused benefits of community involvement and mobilisation. This tension between rigour and community engagement is likely to be enduring.

5 Further Reading

Several applications of the positive deviance approach have been presented as cases and/or referenced throughout this Element. The following further reading is for those who want to find out more about the approach.

- Positive Deviance Collaborative[3] – a website containing tools, manuals, case studies, and publications, and that helps to connect people who are implementing the approach. It predominantly aligns with an international public health approach of positive deviance and covers applications from a variety of counties and settings, including nutrition, education, business, and healthcare.
- Bradley et al.[19] – a summary of the four-stage framework for applying the positive deviance approach in healthcare organisations, and work to improve door-to-balloon times for patients with acute myocardial infarction.
- Lawton et al.[90] – a critique of positive deviance as a new approach to improving patient safety within healthcare organisations.
- Marsh et al.[95] – a commentary introducing the positive deviance approach and describing evidence for its effectiveness.
- Rose and McCullough[67] – a narrative review of the authors' experiences of applying the positive deviance approach in healthcare organisations, including potential applications in healthcare and methodological guidance.

- Baxter et al.[14] – a systematic review of healthcare applications of positive deviance, exploring how positive deviance is defined, the quality of existing applications, and the methods used within them.
- Hibbert and Trubacik[96] – a report detailing how the National Audit for Intermediate Care has used positive deviance to identify and learn from home-based and bed-based intermediate care services in the UK.

Contributors

Rebecca Lawton and Ruth Baxter conceptualised the outline for this Element together. Both authors contributed to the drafting and reviewing of the Element and have approved the final version.

Conflicts of Interest

None.

Acknowledgements

We thank the peer reviewers for their insightful comments and recommendations to improve the Element. A list of peer reviewers is published at www.cambridge.org/IQ-peer-reviewers. We also thank all the staff and patients who have participated in our positive deviance studies.

Funding

This Element was funded by THIS Institute (The Healthcare Improvement Studies Institute, www.thisinstitute.cam.ac.uk). THIS Institute is strengthening the evidence base for improving the quality and safety of healthcare. THIS Institute is supported by a grant to the University of Cambridge from the Health Foundation – an independent charity committed to bringing about better health and healthcare for people in the UK. Our positive deviance studies were funded by the Health Foundation (via a PhD for Improvement Science) and by the NIHR Yorkshire and Humber Collaboration for Leadership in Applied Health Research and Care (CLAHRC – under the Evidence-Based Transformation Theme).

About the Authors

Ruth Baxter is a THIS Institute post-doctoral fellow in the Yorkshire Quality and Safety Research Group. Her research interests include the positive deviance approach, adopting a resilient healthcare and Safety II approach to improving healthcare, and involving patients to improve the quality and safety of healthcare services.

Rebecca Lawton is a health psychologist with two main research interests: patient safety and behaviour change. She is Professor, Psychology of Healthcare, at the University of Leeds, founder member of the Yorkshire Quality and Safety Research Group, and Director of NIHR Yorkshire and Humber Patient Safety Translational Research Centre, with a focus on delivering research that makes healthcare safer.

Creative Commons Licence

References

1. Wray JD. Can we learn from successful mothers? *J Trop Pediatr Environ Child Health* 1972; 18: 279. https://doi.org/10.1093/tropej/18.4.279.

2. Wishik SM, Van Der Vynckt S. The use of nutritional 'positive deviants' to identify approaches for modification of dietary practices. *Am J Public Health* 1976; 66: 38–42. https://doi.org/10.2105/ajph.66.1.38.

3. Positive Deviance Collaborative. https://positivedeviance.org (accessed 12 February 2022).

4. Sternin M, Sternin J, Marsh DL. Rapid, sustained childhood malnutrition alleviation through a positive-deviance approach in rural Vietnam: preliminary findings. In: Wollinka O, Keeley E, Burkhalter BR, Bashir N, editors. *Hearth Nutrition Model: Applications in Haiti, Vietnam, and Bangladesh.* Arlington, VA: BASICS; 1997: 49–62. https://pdf.usaid.gov/pdf_docs/Pnaca868.pdf (accessed 12 February 2022).

5. Sternin M, Sternin J, Marsh D. Scaling up a poverty alleviation and nutrition program in Vietnam. In: Marchione T, editor. *Scaling Up, Scaling Down: Overcoming Malnutrition in Developing Countries.* Amsterdam: Gordon and Breach; 1999: 97–118.

6. Mackintosh UA, Marsh DR, Schroeder DG. Sustained positive deviant child care practices and their effects on child growth in Viet Nam. *Food Nutr Bull* 2002; 23 (suppl 1): 16–25. https://doi.org/10.1177/15648265020234S104.

7. Bisits Bullen PA. The positive deviance/hearth approach to reducing child malnutrition: systematic review. *Trop Med Int Health* 2011; 16: 1354–66. https://doi.org/10.1111/j.1365-3156.2011.02839.x.

8. Nutrition Working Group, Child Survival Collaborations and Resources Group (CORE). *Positive Deviance/Hearth: A Resource Guide for Sustainably Rehabilitating Malnourished Children.* Washington, DC: CORE; 2002. https://coregroup.org/wp-content/uploads/2017/09/Positive-Deviance-Hearth-Resource-Guide.pdf (accessed 12 February 2022).

9. Ahrari M, Kuttab A, Khamis S, et al. Factors associated with successful pregnancy outcomes in upper Egypt: a positive deviance inquiry. *Food Nutr Bull* 2002; 23: 83–8. https://doi.org/10.1177/156482650202300111.

10. Marsh DR, Sternin M, Khadduri R, et al. Identification of model newborn care practices through a positive deviance inquiry to guide behavior-change interventions in Haripur, Pakistan. *Food Nutr Bull* 2002; 4 (suppl 2): 107–16. https://doi.org/10.1177/15648265020234S215.

11. Stuckey HL, Boan J, Kraschnewski JL, et al. Using positive deviance for determining successful weight-control practices. *Qual Health Res* 2011; 21: 563–79. https://doi.org/10.1177/1049732310386623.

12. Masterson JM, Swanson JH. *Female Genital Cutting: Breaking the Silence, Enabling Change*. Washington, DC: International Center for Research on Women and the Centre for Development and Population Activities; 2000. www.icrw.org/wp-content/uploads/2016/10/Female-Genital-Cutting-Breaking-the-Silence-Enabling-Change.pdf (accessed 12 February 2022).

13. Herington MJ, van de Fliert E. Positive deviance in theory and practice: a conceptual review. *Deviant Behav* 2017; 39: 664–78. https://doi.org/10.1080/01639625.2017.1286194.

14. Baxter R, Taylor N, Kellar I, Lawton R. What methods are used to apply positive deviance within healthcare organisations? A systematic review. *BMJ Qual Saf* 2016; 25: 190–201. https://doi.org/10.1136/bmjqs-2015-004386.

15. Positive Deviance Initiative. *Basic Field Guide to the Positive Deviance Approach*. Boston, MA: Tufts University; 2010. https://static1.squarespace.com/static/5a1eeb26fe54ef288246a688/t/5a6eca16c83025f9bac2eeff/1517210135326/FINALguide10072010.pdf (accessed 12 February 2022).

16. Singhal A, Dura L. Positive deviance: a non-normative approach to health and risk messaging. *Oxford Res Encycloped Comm* 2017. https://doi.org/10.1093/acrefore/9780190228613.013.248.

17. Awofeso N, Irwin T, Forrest G. Using positive deviance techniques to improve smoking cessation outcomes in New South Wales prison settings. *Health Promot J Austr* 2008; 19: 72–3. https://citeseerx.ist.psu.edu/viewdoc/download?doi=10.1.1.541.3589&rep=rep1&type=pdf (accessed 12 February 2022).

18. Zaidi Z, Jaffery T, Shahid A, et al. Change in action: using positive deviance to improve student clinical performance. *Adv Health Sci Educ* 2012; 17: 95–105. https://doi.org/10.1007/s10459-011-9301-8.

19. Bradley EH, Curry LA, Ramanadhan S, et al. Research in action: using positive deviance to improve quality of health care. *Implement Sci* 2009; 4: 25. https://doi.org/10.1186/1748-5908-4-25.

20. Bradley EH, Herrin J, Wang Y, et al. Strategies for reducing the door-to-balloon time in acute myocardial infarction. *N Engl J Med* 2006; 355: 2308–20. https://doi.org/10.1056/NEJMsa063117.

21. Bradley EH, Roumanis SA, Radford MJ, et al. Achieving door-to-balloon times that meet quality guidelines: how do successful hospitals do it? *J Am Coll Cardiol* 2005; 46: 1236–41. https://doi.org/10.1016/j.jacc.2005.07.009.

22. Antman EM, Anbe DT, Armstrong PW, et al. ACC/AHA guidelines for the management of patients with ST-elevation myocardial infarction: executive summary. *Circulation* 2004; 110: 588–636. https://doi.org/10.1161/01 .CIR.0000134791.68010.FA.

23. Van de Werf F, Ardissino D, Betriu A, et al. Management of acute myocardial infarction in patients presenting with ST-segment elevation. *Eur Heart J* 2003; 24: 28–66. https://doi.org/10.1016/s0195-668x(02)00618-8.

24. Bradley EH, Byam P, Alpern R, et al. A systems approach to improving rural care in Ethiopia. *PLoS One* 2012; 7: e35042. https://doi.org/10.1371 /journal.pone.0035042.

25. Bradley EH, Curry LA, Spatz ES, et al. Hospital strategies for reducing risk-standardized mortality rates in acute myocardial infarction. *Ann Intern Med* 2012; 56: 618–26. https://doi.org/10.1059/0003-4819-156-9-201205010-00003.

26. Gabbay RA, Friedberg MW, Miller-Day M, et al. A positive deviance approach to understanding key features to improving diabetes care in the medical home. *Ann Fam Med* 2013; 1 (suppl 1): S99–107. https://doi.org /10.1370/afm.1473.

27. Klaiman T, O'Connell K, Stoto M. Local health department public vaccination clinic success during 2009 pH1N1. *J Public Health Manag Pract* 2013; 19: E20–6. https://doi.org/10.1097/PHH.0b013e318269e434.

28. Klaiman T, O'Connell K, Stoto MA. Learning from successful school-based vaccination clinics during 2009 pH1N1. *J Sch Health* 2014; 84: 63–9. https://doi.org/10.1111/josh.12119.

29. Buscell P. The people, the danger and the new deviants. In: Singhal A, Buscell P, Lindberg C, editors. *Inviting Everyone: Healing Healthcare through Positive Deviance.* Bordentown, NJ: PlexusPress; 2010: 1–22. https://utmi ners.utep.edu/asinghal/Books/Singhal-Book-2010-Inviting-Everyone-Healing-healthcare-through-Positive-Deviance.pdf (accessed 12 February 2022).

30. Jain R, Kralovic SM, Evans ME, et al. Veterans Affairs initiative to prevent methicillin-resistant Staphylococcus aureus infections. *N Engl J Med* 2011; 364: 1419–30. https://doi.org/10.1056/NEJMoa1007474.

31. Marra AR, Guastelli LR, de Araujo CMP, et al. Positive deviance: a new strategy for improving hand hygiene compliance. *Infect Control Hosp Epidemiol* 2010; 31: 12–20. https://doi.org/10.1086/649224.

32. Marra AR, Guastelli LR, de Araujo CMP, et al. Positive deviance: a program for sustained improvement in hand hygiene compliance. *Am J Infect Control* 2011; 39: 1–5. https://doi.org/10.1016/j.ajic.2010.05.024.

33. Mannion R, Braithwaite J. False dawns and new horizons in patient safety research and practice. *Int J Health Policy Manag* 2017; 6: 685–9. https://doi.org/10.15171/ijhpm.2017.115.

34. Dixon-Woods M, Martin GP. Does quality improvement improve quality? *Future Hosp J* 2016; 3: 191–4. https://doi.org/10.7861/future hosp.3-3-191.

35. Hollnagel E, Wears RL, Braithwaite J. *From Safety-I to Safety-II: A White Paper*. The Resilient Health Care Net: Published simultaneously by University of Southern Denmark; University of Florida, USA; and Macquarie University, Australia; 2015. www.england.nhs.uk/signuptosaf ety/wp-content/uploads/sites/16/2015/10/safety-1-safety-2-whte-papr.pdf (accessed 12 February 2022).

36. Hollnagel E, Braithwaite J, Wears RL. *Resilient Health Care.* Surrey: Ashgate; 2013.

37. Learning from Excellence. https://learningfromexcellence.com (accessed 12 February 2022).

38. Appreciating People. How Appreciative Inquiry Can Help You. www .appreciatingpeople.co.uk/how-ai-can-help-you (accessed 12 February 2022).

39. Kelly N, Blake S, Plunkett A. Learning from excellence in healthcare: a new approach to incident reporting. *Arch Dis Child* 2016; 101: 788–91. https://doi.org/10.1136/archdischild-2015-310021.

40. Learning from Excellence. Is Learning from Excellence 'Safety-II'? 2017. https://learningfromexcellence.com/how-do-you-do-safety-ii (accessed 12 February 2022).

41. Richer M, Ritchie J, Marchionni C. Appreciative inquiry in health care. *Br J Healthc Manage* 2010; 16: 164–72. https://doi.org/10.12968/bjhc .2010.16.4.47399.

42. Trajkovski S, Schmied V, Vickers M, Jackson D. Using appreciative inquiry to transform health care. *Contemp Nurse* 2013; 45: 95–100. https://doi.org/10.5172/conu.2013.45.1.95.

43. Lilford R, Mohammed MA, Spiegelhalter D, Thomson R. Use and misuse of process and outcome data in managing performance of acute medical care: avoiding institutional stigma. *Lancet* 2004; 363: 1147–54. https://doi .org/10.1016/S0140-6736(04)15901-1.

44. Dixon-Woods M, Leslie M, Bion J, Tarrant C. What counts? An ethnographic study of infection data reported to a patient safety program. *Milbank Q* 2012; 90: 548–91. https://doi.org/10.1111/j.1468-0009 .2012.00674.x.

45. Vincent C, Burnett S, Carthey J. *The Measurement and Monitoring of Safety: Drawing Together Academic Evidence and Practical Experience*

to Produce a Framework for Safety Measurement and Monitoring. London: The Health Foundation; 2013. www.health.org.uk/publications/the-measurement-and-monitoring-of-safety (accessed 12 February 2022).

46. Woodcock T, Liberati EG, Dixon-Woods M. A mixed-methods study of challenges experienced by clinical teams in measuring improvement. *BMJ Qual Saf* 2021; 30: 106–15. https://doi.org/10.1136/bmjqs-2018-009048.

47. Pronovost PJ, Nolan T, Zeger S, Miller M, Rubin H. How can clinicians measure safety and quality in acute care? *Lancet* 2004; 363: 1061–7. https://doi.org/10.1016/S0140-6736(04)15843-1.

48. O'Hara JK, Grasic K, Gutacker N, et al. Identifying positive deviants in healthcare quality and safety: a mixed methods study. *J R Soc Med* 2018; 111: 276–91. https://doi.org/10.1177/0141076818772230.

49. The Royal College of Surgeons of England. Surgical Outcomes. www.rcseng.ac.uk/patient-care/surgical-staff-and-regulation/surgical-outcomes (accessed 12 February 2022).

50. Healthcare Quality Improvement Partnership. The National Clinical Audit Programme. www.hqip.org.uk/a-z-of-nca/#.Xqw6gp5KjIU (accessed 12 February 2022).

51. Austin JM, Jha AK, Romano PS, et al. National hospital ratings systems share few common scores and may generate confusion instead of clarity. *Health Aff* 2015; 34: 423–30. https://doi.org/10.1377/hlthaff.2014.0201.

52. Jacobson B, Mindell J, McKee M. Hospital mortality league tables: question what they tell you – and how useful they are. *BMJ* 2003; 326: 777–8. https://doi.org/10.1136/bmj.326.7393.777.

53. Rothberg MB, Morsi E, Benjamin EM, Pekow PS, Lindenauer PK. Choosing the best hospital: the limitations of public quality reporting. *Health Aff (Millwood)* 2008; 27: 1680–7. https://doi.org/10.1377/hlthaff.27.6.1680.

54. Baxter R, Taylor N, Kellar I, et al. Identifying positively deviant elderly medical wards using routinely collected NHS safety thermometer data: an observational study. *BMJ Open* 2018; 8: e020219. https://doi.org/10.1136/bmjopen-2017-020219.

55. Benneyan JC, Lloyd RC, Plsek PE. Statistical process control as a tool for research and healthcare improvement. *Qual Saf Health Care* 2003; 12: 458–64. https://doi.org/10.1136/qhc.12.6.458.

56. Mohammed MA, Worthington P, Woodall WH. Plotting basic control charts: tutorial notes for healthcare practitioners. *Qual Saf Health Care* 2008; 17: 137–45. https://doi.org/10.1136/qshc.2004.012047.

57. Marshall T, Mohammed MA, Rouse A. A randomized controlled trial of league tables and control charts as aids to health service decision-making.

Int J Qual Health Care 2004; 16: 309–15. https://doi.org/10.1093/intqhc/mzh054.

58. Mohammed MA. Statistical process control. In: Dixon-Woods M, Brown K, Marjanovic S, et al., editors. *Elements of Improving Quality and Safety in Healthcare*. Cambridge: Cambridge University Press; forthcoming.

59. Griffith JR, Fear KM, Lammers E, et al. A positive deviance perspective on hospital knowledge management: analysis of Baldrige Award recipients 2002–2008. *J Healthc Manag* 2013; 58: 187–203. https://doi.org/10.1097/00115514-201305000-00007.

60. Sheard L, Jackson C, Lawton R. How is success achieved by individuals innovating for patient safety and quality in the NHS? *BMC Health Serv Res* 2017; 17: 640. https://doi.org/10.1186/s12913-017-2589-1.

61. Marra AR, Noritomi DT, Westheimer Cavalcante AJ, et al. A multicenter study using positive deviance for improving hand hygiene compliance. *Am J Infect Control* 2013; 41: 984–8. https://doi.org/10.1016/j.ajic.2013.05.013.

62. Baxter R, Taylor N, Kellar I, Lawton R. Learning from positively deviant wards to improve patient safety: an observational study protocol. *BMJ Open* 2015; 5: e009650. https://doi.org/10.1136/bmjopen-2015-009650.

63. Baxter R, Taylor N, Kellar I, Lawton R. A qualitative positive deviance study to explore exceptionally safe care on medical wards for older people. *BMJ Qual Saf* 2019; 28: 618–26. https://doi.org/10.1136/bmjqs-2018-008023.

64. Kraschnewski JL, Sciamanna CN, Pollak KI, Stuckey HL, Sherwood NE. The epidemiology of weight counseling for adults in the United States: a case of positive deviance. *Int J Obes (Lond)* 2013; 37: 751–3. https://doi.org/10.1038/ijo.2012.113.

65. Rose AJ, Petrakis BA, Callahan P, et al. Organizational characteristics of high- and low-performing anticoagulation clinics in the Veterans Health Administration. *Health Serv Res* 2012; 47: 1541–60. https://doi.org/10.1111/j.1475-6773.2011.01377.x.

66. Davidoff F, Dixon-Woods M, Leviton L, Michie S. Demystifying theory and its use in improvement. *BMJ Qual Saf* 2015; 24: 228–38. https://doi.org/10.1136/bmjqs-2014-003627.

67. Rose AJ, McCullough MB. A practical guide to using the positive deviance method in health services research. *Health Serv Res* 2017; 52: 1207–22. https://doi.org/10.1111/1475-6773.12524.

68. Lawton R, McEachan RR, Giles SJ, et al. Development of an evidence-based framework of factors contributing to patient safety incidents in hospital settings: a systematic review. *BMJ Qual Saf* 2012; 21: 369–80. https://doi.org/10.1136/bmjqs-2011-000443.

69. National Patient Safety Agency. Manchester Patient Safety Framework (MaPSaF). 2006. https://webarchive.nationalarchives.gov.uk/ukgwa/20171030124256/http://www.nrls.npsa.nhs.uk/resources/?EntryId45=59796 (accessed 12 February 2022).

70. Michie S, van Stralen M, West R. The behaviour change wheel: a new method for characterising and designing behaviour change interventions. *Implement Sci* 2011; 6: 42. https://doi.org/10.1186/1748-5908-6-42.

71. Rycroft-Malone J, Harvey G, Seers K, et al. An exploration of the factors that influence the implementation of evidence into practice. *J Clin Nurs* 2004; 13: 913–24. https://doi.org/10.1111/j.1365-2702.2004.01007.x.

72. Liberati EG, Tarrant C, Willars J, et al. How to be a very safe maternity unit: an ethnographic study. *Soc Sci Med* 2019; 223: 64–72. https://doi.org/10.1016/j.socscimed.2019.01.035.

73. Curry LA, Spatz E, Cherlin E, et al. What distinguishes top-performing hospitals in acute myocardial infarction mortality rates? A qualitative study. *Ann Intern Med* 2011; 154: 384–90. https://doi.org/10.7326/0003-4819-154-6-201103150-00003.

74. Hughes L, Sheard L, Pinkney L, Lawton RL. Excellence in elective hip and knee surgery: what does it look like? A positive deviance approach. *J Health Serv Res Policy* 2020; 25: 5–12. https://doi.org/10.1177/1355819619867350.

75. Maryland Patient Safety Centre. Field Guide 2007. https://static1.squarespace.com/static/5a1eeb26fe54ef288246a688/t/5ac7d891aa4a996d8d80ff9d/1523046565385/Healthcare_Manual (accessed 12 February 2022).

76. Lindberg C, Downham G, Buscell P, et al. Embracing collaboration: a novel strategy for reducing bloodstream infections in outpatient hemodialysis centers. *Am J Infect Control* 2013; 41: 513–19. https://doi.org/10.1016/j.ajic.2012.07.015.

77. Singhal A, Buscell P. Actions speak louder than MRSA at Billings clinic. In: Singhal A, Buscell P, Lindberg C, editors. *Inviting Everyone: Healing Healthcare through Positive Deviance*. Bordentown, NJ: PlexusPress; 2010: 95–123. https://utminers.utep.edu/asinghal/Books/Singhal-Book-2010-Inviting-Everyone-Healing-healthcare-through-Positive-Deviance.pdf (accessed 12 February 2022).

78. Michie S, Richardson M, Johnston M, et al. The behavior change technique taxonomy (v1) of 93 hierarchically clustered techniques: building an international consensus for the reporting of behavior change interventions. *Ann Behav Med* 2013; 46: 81–95. https://doi.org/10.1007/s12160-013-9486-6.

79. Singhal A, Greiner K. Small solutions and big rewards: MRSA prevention at the Pittsburgh Veterans hospitals. In: Singhal A, Buscell P, Lindberg C,

editors. *Inviting Everyone: Healing Healthcare through Positive Deviance.* Bordentown, NJ: PlexusPress; 2010: 47–67. https://utminers.utep.edu/asin ghal/Books/Singhal-Book-2010-Inviting-Everyone-Healing-healthcare-through-Positive-Deviance.pdf (accessed 12 February 2022).

80. Singhal A, McCandless K, Buscell P, Lindberg C. Spanning silos and spurring conversations: positive deviance for reducing infection in hospitals. *Performance* 2009; 2: 78–83. http://utminers.utep.edu/asinghal/ Articles%20and%20Chapters/Journal%20Articles/Singhal-McCandless-Buscell-Lindberg-MRSA-Performance_2009-Article-EandY.pdf (accessed 12 February 2022).

81. Krumholz HM, Bradley EH, Nallamothu BK, et al. A campaign to improve the timeliness of primary percutaneous coronary intervention: door-to-balloon: an alliance for quality. *JACC Cardiovasc Interv* 2008; 1: 97–104. https://doi.org/10.1016/j.jcin.2007.10.006.

82. Sreeramoju P, Dura L, Fernandez ME, et al. Using a positive deviance approach to influence the culture of patient safety related to infection prevention. *Open Forum Infect Dis* 2018; 5: ofy231. https://doi.org/10 .1093/ofid/ofy231.

83. Bate P, Robert G, Fulop N, Øvretveit J, Dixon-Woods M. *Perspectives on Context: A Selection of Essays Considering the Role of Context in Successful Quality Improvement.* London: The Health Foundation; 2014. www .health.org.uk/publications/perspectives-on-context (accessed 12 February 2022).

84. Bion J, Richardson A, Hibbert P, et al. 'Matching Michigan': a 2-year stepped interventional programme to minimise central venous catheter-blood stream infections in intensive care units in England. *BMJ Qual Saf* 2013; 22: 110–23. https://doi.org/10.1136/bmjqs-2012-001325.

85. Dixon-Woods M, Leslie M, Tarrant C, Bion J. Explaining Matching Michigan: an ethnographic study of a patient safety program. *Implement Sci* 2013; 8: 70. https://doi.org/10.1186/1748-5908-8-70.

86. Kim YM, Heerey M, Kols A. Factors that enable nurse-patient communi-cation in a family planning context: a positive deviance study. *Int J Nurs Stud* 2008; 45: 1411–21. https://doi.org/10.1016/j.ijnurstu.2008.01.002.

87. Martin G, Dixon-Woods M. Collaboration-based approaches. In: Dixon-Woods M, Brown K, Marjanovic S, et al., editors. *Elements of Improving Quality and Safety in Healthcare.* Cambridge: Cambridge University Press; 2022. https://doi.org/10.1017/9781009236867.

88. Mannion R. Making culture change happen. In: Dixon-Woods M, Brown K, Marjanovic S, et al., editors. *Elements of Improving Quality*

and Safety in Healthcare. Cambridge: Cambridge University Press; 2022. https://doi.org/10.1017/9781009236935.

89. Papoutsi C, Greenhalgh T, Marjanovic S. Approaches to spread, scale-up, and sustainability. In: Dixon-Woods M, Brown K, Marjanovic S, et al., editors. *Elements of Improving Quality and Safety in Healthcare.* Cambridge: Cambridge University Press; forthcoming.

90. Lawton R, Taylor N, Clay-Williams R, Braithwaite J. Positive deviance: a different approach to achieving patient safety. *BMJ Qual Saf* 2014; 23: 880–3. https://doi.org/10.1136/bmjqs-2014-003115.

91. Ivers N, Foy R. Audit, feedback, and behaviour change. In: Dixon-Woods M, Brown K, Marjanovic S, et al., editors. *Elements of Improving Quality and Safety in Healthcare.* Cambridge: Cambridge University Press; forthcoming.

92. Cohen R, Gesser-Edelsburg A, Singhal A, Benenson S, Moses AE. Deconstruction of central line insertion guidelines based on the positive deviance approach-reducing gaps between guidelines and implementation: a qualitative ethnographic research. *PLoS One* 2019; 14: e0222608. https://doi.org/10.1371/journal.pone.0222608.

93. Plsek PE, Greenhalgh T. The challenge of complexity in health care. *BMJ* 2001; 323: 625–8. https://doi.org/10.1136/bmj.323.7313.625.

94. Lindberg C, Schneider M. Combating infections at Maine Medical Center: insights into complexity-informed leadership from positive deviance. *Leadership* 2013; 9: 229–53. https://doi.org/10.1177/1742715012468784.

95. Marsh DR, Schroeder DG, Dearden KA, Sternin J, Sternin M. The power of positive deviance. *BMJ* 2004; 329: 1177–9. https://doi.org/10.1136/bmj.329.7475.1177.

96. Hibbert D, Trubacik T. *Positive Deviance in Intermediate Care Services.* UK: National Audit of Intermediate Care, NHS Benchmarking Unit; 2019. https://s3.eu-west-2.amazonaws.com/nhsbn-static/NAIC%20(Providers)/2018/Positive%20deviance%20inintermediate%20care%20services%20FINAL.pdf (accessed 12 February 2022).

Cambridge Elements ☰

Improving Quality and Safety in Healthcare

Editors-in-Chief

Mary Dixon-Woods

THIS Institute (The Healthcare Improvement Studies Institute)

Mary is Director of THIS Institute and is the Health Foundation Professor of Healthcare Improvement Studies in the Department of Public Health and Primary Care at the University of Cambridge. Mary leads a programme of research focused on healthcare improvement, healthcare ethics, and methodological innovation in studying healthcare.

Graham Martin

THIS Institute (The Healthcare Improvement Studies Institute)

Graham is Director of Research at THIS Institute, leading applied research programmes and contributing to the institute's strategy and development. His research interests are in the organisation and delivery of healthcare, and particularly the role of professionals, managers, and patients and the public in efforts at organisational change.

Executive Editor

Katrina Brown

THIS Institute (The Healthcare Improvement Studies Institute)

Katrina is Communications Manager at THIS Institute, providing editorial expertise to maximise the impact of THIS Institute's research findings. She managed the project to produce the series.

Editorial Team

Sonja Marjanovic

RAND Europe

Sonja is Director of RAND Europe's healthcare innovation, industry, and policy research. Her work provides decision-makers with evidence and insights to support innovation and improvement in healthcare systems, and to support the translation of innovation into societal benefits for healthcare services and population health.

Tom Ling

RAND Europe

Tom is Head of Evaluation at RAND Europe and President of the European Evaluation Society, leading evaluations and applied research focused on the key challenges facing health services. His current health portfolio includes evaluations of the innovation landscape, quality improvement, communities of practice, patient flow, and service transformation.

Ellen Perry

THIS Institute (The Healthcare Improvement Studies Institute)

Ellen supported the production of the series during 2020–21.

About the Series

The past decade has seen enormous growth in both activity and research on improvement in healthcare. This series offers a comprehensive and authoritative set of overviews of the different improvement approaches available, exploring the thinking behind them, examining evidence for each approach, and identifying areas of debate.

Cambridge Elements $^{\equiv}$

Improving Quality and Safety in Healthcare

Elements in the Series

Collaboration-Based Approaches
Graham Martin and Mary Dixon-Woods

Co-Producing and Co-Designing
Glenn Robert, Louise Locock, Oli Williams, Jocelyn Cornwell, Sara Donetto, and Joanna Goodrich

The Positive Deviance Approach
Ruth Baxter and Rebecca Lawton

A full series listing is available at: www.cambridge.org/IQ

Printed in the United States
by Baker & Taylor Publisher Services